The Ultimate Vegetarian Savory Dish Cooking Guide

Delicious Savory Vegetarian Recipes For Beginners

Riley Bloom

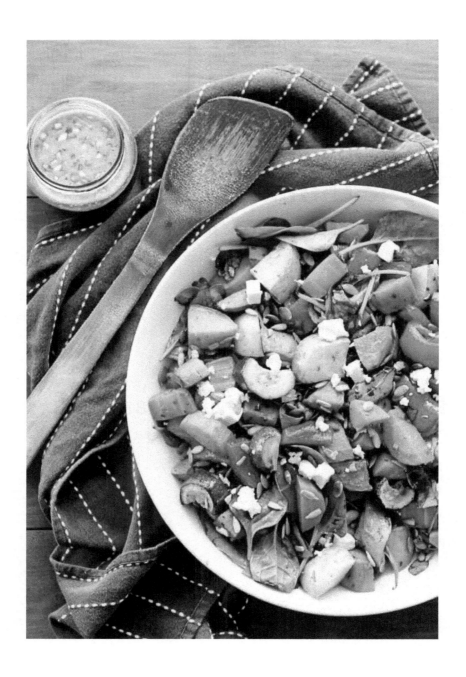

Table of contents

5

Grilled Beetroots and Broccolini

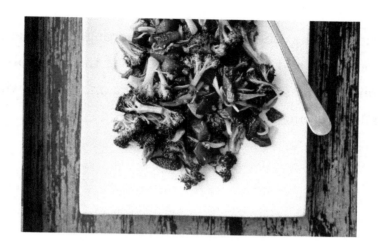

Ingredients

2 beetroots, peeled and sliced lengthwise

1 large red onion, cut into 1/2 inch thick rounds

1/3 cup Italian parsley or basil, finely chopped

10 Broccolini Florets

10 pcs. Brussel Sprouts

Dressing Ingredients

6 tbsp. olive oil

3 dashes of Tabasco hot sauce

Sea salt, to taste 3 tbsp.

white wine vinegar 1 tsp.

Directions:

<u>Egg-free mayonnaise</u>

Combine all of the dressing ingredients thoroughly. Preheat your grill to low heat and grease the grates. Layer the vegetables grill for 12 minutes per side, until tender flipping once. Brush with the marinade/ dressing ingredients

Grilled Artichokes and Mustard Greens

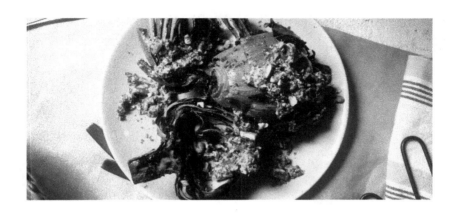

Ingredients

1 pc. Artichoke

1 bunch of mustard greens

1/3 cup Italian parsley or basil, finely chopped

Dressing Ingredients

6 tbsp. extra virgin olive oil

Sea salt, to taste 3 tbsp.

apple cider vinegar 1 tbsp.

honey 1 tsp.

Directions:

Egg-free mayonnaise

Combine all of the dressing ingredients thoroughly. Preheat your grill to low heat and grease the grates. Layer the vegetables grill for 12 minutes per side, until tender flipping once. Brush with the marinade/ dressing ingredients

Grilled Beets and Swiss Chard

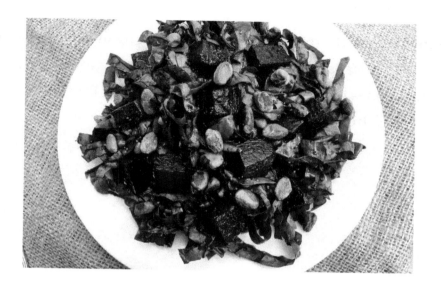

Ingredients

5 pcs. Beets

1 bunch of swiss chard

4 large Tomatoes, sliced thick

1/3 cup Italian parsley or basil, finely chopped

Dressing Ingredients:

6 tbsp. extra virgin olive oil

1 tsp. onion powder

Sea salt, to taste

3 tbsp. distilled white vinegar 1 tsp.

Directions:

<u>Dijon mustard</u>

Combine all of the dressing ingredients thoroughly. Preheat your grill to low heat and grease the grates. Layer the vegetables grill for 12 minutes per side, until tender flipping once. Brush with the marinade/ dressing ingredients

Grilled Baby Corn and Winter Squash

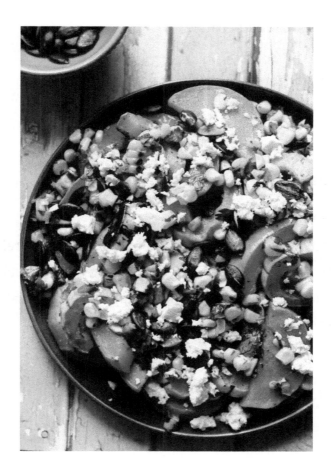

Ingredients

10 pcs. baby corn

1 winter squash, peeled and sliced lengthwise

1 large red onion, cut into 1/2 inch thick rounds

1/3 cup Italian parsley or basil, finely chopped

Dressing Ingredients

6 tbsp. olive oil

3 dashes of Tabasco hot sauce

Sea salt, to taste 3 tbsp.

white wine vinegar 1 tsp.

Directions:

Egg-free mayonnaise

Combine all of the dressing ingredients thoroughly. Preheat your grill to low heat and grease the grates. Layer the vegetables grill for 12 minutes per side, until tender flipping once. Brush with the marinade/ dressing ingredients

Grilled Beets and Asparagus

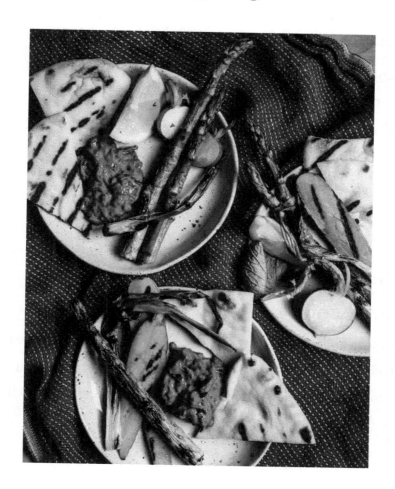

Ingredients

5 pcs. Beets

10 pcs. Asparagus

1 winter squash, peeled and sliced lengthwise

4 large Tomatoes, sliced thick

1 lb green bell peppers, sliced into wide strips

1 large red onion, cut into 1/2 inch thick rounds

1/3 cup Italian parsley or basil, finely chopped

<u>Dressing Ingredients</u>

6 tbsp. extra virgin olive oil

Sea salt, to taste 3 tbsp.

apple cider vinegar 1 tbsp.

honey 1 tsp.

Directions:

<u>Egg-free mayonnaise</u>

Combine all of the dressing ingredients thoroughly. Preheat your grill to low heat and grease the grates. Layer the vegetables grill for 12 minutes per side, until tender flipping once. Brush with the marinade/ dressing ingredients

Grilled Artichoke

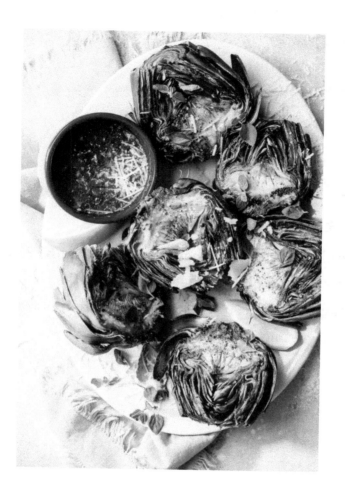

Ingredients

1 pc. Artichoke

1/3 cup Italian parsley or basil, finely chopped

Dressing Ingredients:

6 tbsp. extra virgin olive oil

1 tsp. onion powder

Sea salt, to taste 3 tbsp.

distilled white vinegar 1 tsp.

Directions:

Dijon mustard

Combine all of the dressing ingredients thoroughly. Preheat your grill to low heat and grease the grates. Layer the vegetables grill for 12 minutes per side, until tender flipping once. Brush with the marinade/ dressing ingredients

Grilled Summer Squash Cabbage and Romaine Lettuce

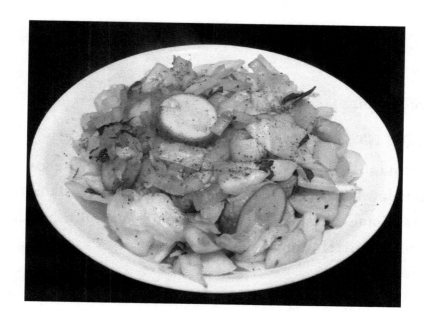

Ingredients

1 medium Cabbage sliced

1 summer squash, peeled and sliced lengthwise

4 large Tomatoes, sliced thick

1 large red onion, cut into 1/2 inch thick rounds

1/3 cup Italian parsley or basil, finely chopped

Dressing Ingredients

6 tbsp. olive oil

3 dashes of Tabasco hot sauce

Sea salt, to taste

3 tbsp.

white wine vinegar 1 tsp.

Directions:

<u>Egg-free mayonnaise</u>

Combine all of the dressing ingredients thoroughly. Preheat your grill to low heat and grease the grates. Layer the vegetables grill for 12 minutes per side, until tender flipping once. Brush with the marinade/ dressing ingredients

Grilled Rutabaga Baby Carrots and Brussels Sprouts

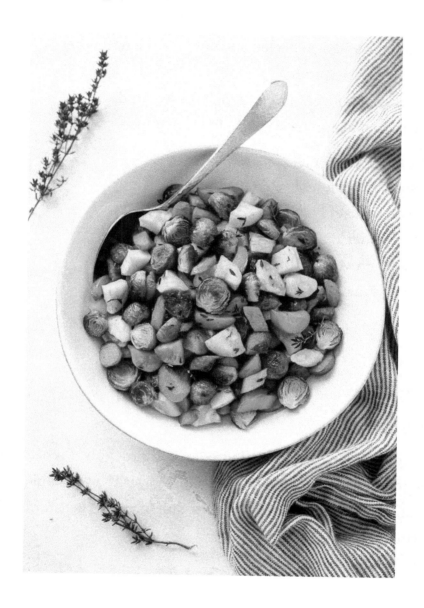

Ingredients

8 pcs. baby carrots

1 lb green bell peppers, sliced into wide strips

1 medium Rutabaga, peeled and cut in half lengthwise

10 pcs. Brussel Sprouts

1 large red onion, cut into 1/2 inch thick rounds

1/3 cup Italian parsley or basil, finely chopped

Dressing Ingredients

6 tbsp. extra virgin olive oil

Sea salt, to taste 1 tsp.

onion powder 1/2 tsp.

Herbs de Provence 3 tbsp.

white vinegar 1 tsp.

Directions:

Dijon mustard

Combine all of the dressing ingredients thoroughly. Preheat your grill to low heat and grease the grates. Layer the vegetables grill for 12 minutes per side, until tender flipping once. Brush with the marinade/ dressing ingredients

Grilled Kale Beets and Carrots

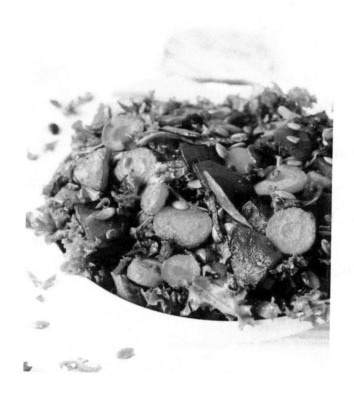

Ingredients

1 bunch of Kale

5 pcs. Beets

2 medium Carrots, cut lengthwise and cut in half

4 large Tomatoes, sliced thick

1 large red onion, cut into 1/2 inch thick rounds

1/3 cup Italian parsley or basil, finely chopped

<u>Dressing Ingredients:</u>

6 tbsp. extra virgin olive oil

1 tsp. onion powder

Sea salt, to taste 3 tbsp.

distilled white vinegar 1 tsp.

Directions:

<u>Dijon mustard</u>

Combine all of the dressing ingredients thoroughly. Preheat your grill to low heat and grease the grates. Layer the vegetables grill for 12 minutes per side, until tender flipping once. Brush with the marinade/ dressing ingredients

Grilled Turnip Greens Okra and Red Onion

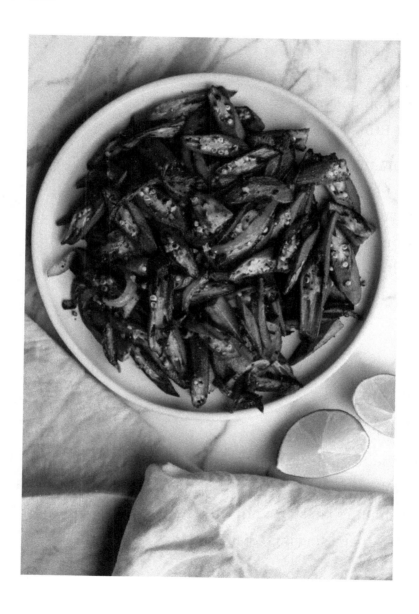

Ingredients

1 bunch of turnip greens

10 pcs. Okra

1 large red onion, cut into 1/2 inch thick rounds

1/3 cup Italian parsley or basil, finely chopped

10 Broccolini Florets

10 pcs. Brussel Sprouts

Dressing Ingredients

6 tbsp. olive oil

1 tsp. garlic powder

1 tsp. onion powder

Sea salt, to taste 3 tbsp.

white wine vinegar 1 tsp.

Directions:

English mustard

Combine all of the dressing ingredients thoroughly. Preheat your grill to low heat and grease the grates. Layer the vegetables grill for 12 minutes per side, until tender flipping once. Brush with the marinade/ dressing ingredients

Grilled Collard Greens Artichoke , Carrots and Kale

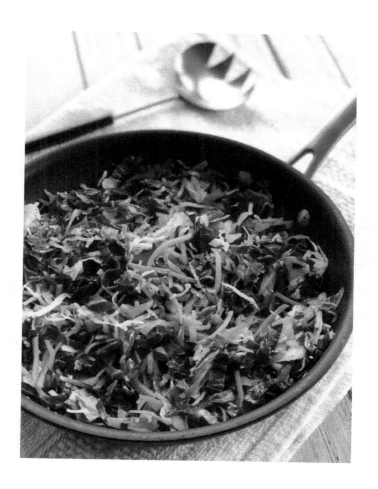

Ingredients

1 pc. Artichoke

1 bunch of Kale

1 bunch of collard greens

1 large white onion, cut into 1/2-inch slices

Dressing Ingredients

6 tbsp. olive oil

3 dashes of Tabasco hot sauce

Sea salt, to taste 3 tbsp.

white wine vinegar 1 tsp.

Directions:

Egg-free mayonnaise

Combine all of the dressing ingredients thoroughly. Preheat your grill to low heat and grease the grates. Layer the vegetables grill for 12 minutes per side, until tender flipping once. Brush with the marinade/ dressing ingredients

Grilled Water Chestnuts and Asparagus

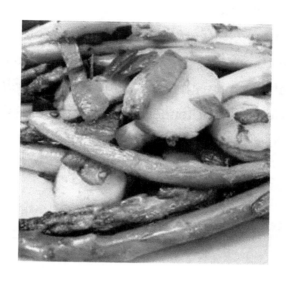

Ingredients

2 teaspoons finely grated lemon zest

2 tablespoon fresh lemon juice

1 tablespoon English mustard

¼ cup extra virgin olive oil, plus more Sea salt, freshly ground
pepper

2 large bunches thick asparagus, trimmed

1/2 cup canned water chestnuts

2 bunches spring onions, halved if large

Directions:

Preheat grill for medium-high heat. Combine lemon zest, lemon juice, mustard, and ¼ cup oil in a bowl Season with salt and pepper. Place the asparagus and spring onions on a pan and drizzle with oil. Season with sea salt and pepper. Grill for about 4 minutes per side or until tender. Sprinkle the dressing over the grilled vegetables.

Grilled Butternut Squash with Chipotle

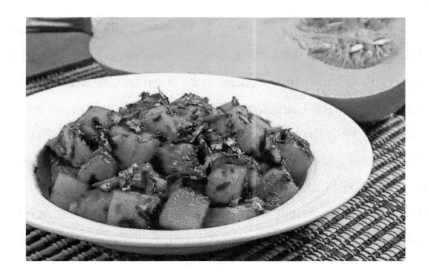

Ingredients

½ cup olive oil, plus more for grill

1 butternut squash, peeled and sliced lengthwise

2 canned chipotle chilies in adobo, finely chopped, plus

3 tablespoons adobo sauce

8 garlic cloves, finely grated

6 tablespoons red wine vinegar

3 tablespoons honey

2 tablespoons kosher salt

2 tablespoons smoked paprika

1 tablespoon dried oregano Lemon wedges (for serving)

Directions:

Prepare your grill for medium-low heat and oil the grates. Slice the cauliflower into 4 equal parts. Add the chilies, adobo sauce, garlic, vinegar, molasses, salt, paprika, oregano, and remaining ½ cup olive oil in a medium bowl to combine. Brush this sauce on one side of each cauliflower steak and place steaks, sauce side down, on grill. Brush the second side with sauce. Grill the cauliflower until tender for 7–8 minutes. Drizzle the cooked side with sauce Grill until second side softens, 7–8 minutes. Move to indirect heat, and brush with the sauce. C Grill until tender. This takes about 20 minutes. Serve with lemon wedges.

Grilled Beetroots with Poblano Chilies

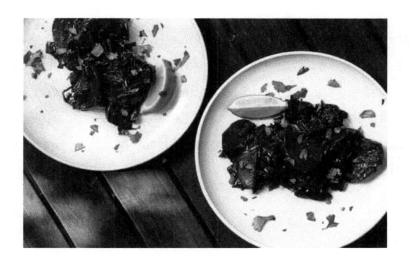

Ingredients

Olive oil (for grill)

2 tablespoons fresh lemon juice

¾ teaspoon hot sauce (such as Frank's)

Sea salt

2 beetroots, peeled and sliced lengthwise

2 small poblano chilies

3 tablespoons extra virgin olive oil

2 scallions, chopped

Preheat your grill for medium heat

Oil the grate.

Directions:

Combine the lime juice and hot sauce in a bowl and season with salt. Grill the corn with the husk on and chilies. Turn frequently, until corn husk is charred and chilies are lightly charred Drizzle corn with olive oil. Cut the kernels. Remove the seeds from chilies and chop finely. Combine the corn with the scallions Season with sea salt.

Grilled Portbello Mushrooms with Almond Lemon Dip

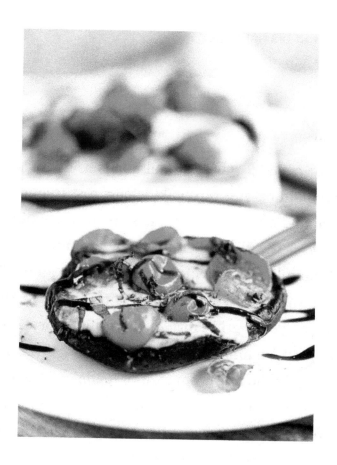

Ingredients

1½ cups whole blanched almonds

1 tablespoon fresh lemon juice

4 tablespoons extra virgin olive oil, divided

1 tablespoon plus 2 teaspoons sherry vinegar, divided

Sea salt

1 pound fresh Portobello mushrooms, stems trimmed, halved lengthwise

Freshly ground black pepper

Directions:

Preheat your oven to 350°. Set 6 almonds aside for garnishing. Toast the remaining nuts on a baking pan, toss frequently. Roast until golden and aromatic. This takes about 8–10 minutes. In a blender process the almonds until finely ground. Add in lemon juice, 2 Tbsp. oil, 1 Tbsp. vinegar, and ½ cup water. Blend by adding more water until dip becomes fairly smooth Season with salt. Prepare your grill for medium-high heat. Combine mushrooms and remaining 2 Tbsp. oil in a bowl. Season with salt and pepper. Grill the mushrooms until tender and charred. This takes about 5 minutes. Return the mushrooms to the bowl and combine with the remaining 2 tsp. vinegar. Serve mushrooms with the dip and garnish with almonds.

Grilled Smoky Butternut Squash with Vegan Yogurt

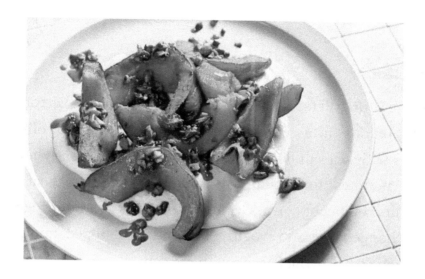

Ingredients

1 butternut squash, peeled and sliced lengthwise

2 bunches scallions, tops trimmed, halved lengthwise

4 tablespoons extra virgin olive oil, divided

Sea salt

1 teaspoon cumin seeds

1 Serrano chili, finely chopped, plus more sliced for serving

1 cup plain yogurt

3 tbsp. fresh lime juice

2 tablespoons chopped mint, plus leaves for serving

A spice mill or mortar and pestle

Directions:

Prepare your grill for medium-low heat. Combine the carrots and spring onions on a rimmed baking pan with 2 Tbsp. olive oil Season with sea salt. Grill and cover, turning frequently tender, 15–20 minutes. toast cumin in a pan over medium heat until fragrant. Let it cool down. Grind and mix this in a bowl together with chopped Serrano, yogurt, lime juice, chopped mint, and remaining 2 Tbsp. oil. Season with sea salt.

Grilled Cauliflower Broccoli and Asparagus

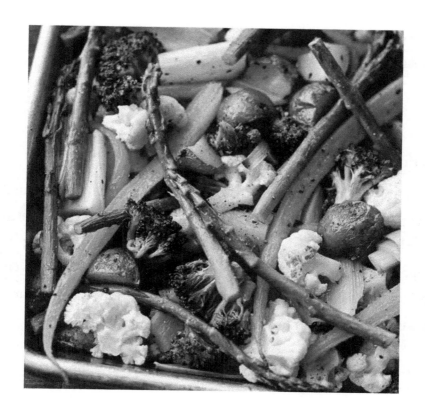

Ingredients

Cauliflower Broccoli Asparagus

½ cup extra virgin olive oil

1/2 tsp Italian seasoning

Sea salt & pepper to taste

1/2 fresh lemon Wash, drain and cut veggies.

For the Marinade combine:

Olive oil (1/8 cup)

Tuscan Herb

Olive oil (1/8 cup) Italian seasoning (1/2 tsp.)

Sea salt & pepper to taste.

Directions:

Marinate the cauliflower & broccoli florets with the marinade ingredients for 45 minutes in a zip top bag at room temperature. Sprinkle the olive oil on the asparagus. Season with 3/4 tsp. pepper and some Sea salt to taste Heat the grill to medium Grill until vegetables become tender and crisp. Squeeze the lemon juice over the vegetables

Grilled Spiraled Eggplants with Tomatoes

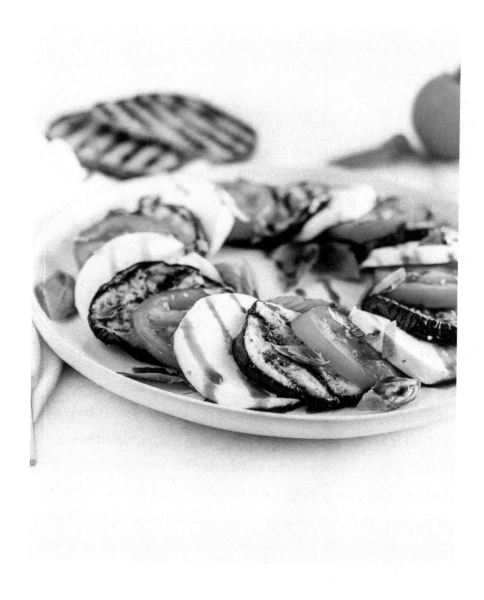

Ingredients

<u>Filling Ingredients</u>

1 1/2 cups yogurt

1/2 cup finely pecorino romano cheese

1 tablespoon fresh juice from

1 lemon

2 tsp. finely minced fresh oregano

1 teaspoon finely minced fresh mint

1 teaspoon finely minced fresh dill

1 teaspoon minced garlic (about

1 medium clove)

Sea salt and Freshly ground black pepper

Directions:

<u>For the Eggplant Rolls:</u>

2 large eggplants, ends trimmed and cut lengthwise into 1/4-inch slices 1/3 cup extra-virgin olive oil 3 Roma tomatoes, stemmed, cored, and cut into 1/4-inch dice 1 English cucumber, seeded and cut into 1/4-inch dice Sea salt and Freshly ground black pepper. Preheat your grill heat to medium-high. Combine the filling ingredients Drizzle eggplants with olive oil, salt and pepper. Grill eggplants on medium heat for 2 ½ min. each side.

Let it cool down for 4 min. Spread the filling ingredients over each eggplant and top with tomatoes and cucumbers. Roll the eggplants into spirals.

Shishito Peppers Skewers With Teriyaki Glaze Recipe

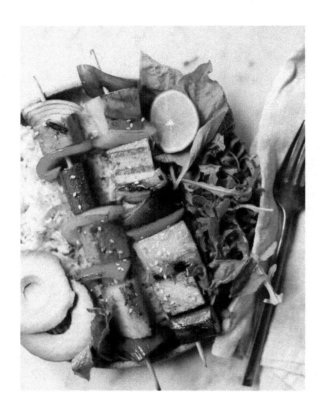

Ingredients

1 pound shishito peppers

Sea salt

Freshly ground black pepper

1/4 cup teriyaki sauce

Skewer the peppers onto sets of 2 skewers, keeping each of them about 1 inch apart to make them easier to flip.

Directions:

Preheat your grill to medium-high. Grill each pepper until charred on one side, about 2 minutes. Flip peppers and grill on the other side, about 2 minutes longer. Season with salt and pepper. Brush with teriyaki sauce.

Avocado Lima Beans and Tomato Bowl

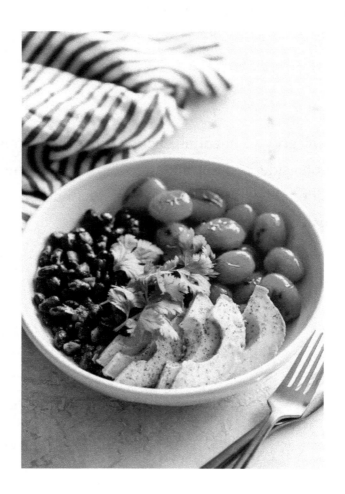

Ingredients

1/2 cup Lima Beans, warmed

1 teaspoon extra-virgin olive oil

1/2 cup Roma tomatoes

1/4 cup fresh corn kernels (from 1 ear)

1/2 medium-sized ripe avocado, thinly sliced

1 medium radish, very thinly sliced

2 tablespoons fresh cilantro leaves

1/2 medium-sized ripe

Sea salt

1/8 teaspoon black pepper

Directions:

Heat the skillet over medium high heat. Add oil to the pan. Add tomatoes to the oil and cook until tender but charred for about 3 minutes. Set the tomatoes beside the beans in a large bowl. Cook the corn and cook for 2 ½ min. Place the corn next to the tomatoes. Add avocado, radish, and cilantro. Season with salt and pepper.

Brussels Tempeh with Soy Dressing

Ingredients

2 tablespoons sesame oil, divided

4 ounces tempeh, thinly sliced

4 teaspoons

l soy sauce

2 teaspoons sherry vinegar

1/8 teaspoon Sea salt

2 tablespoons chopped fresh cilantro, divided

2 beetroots, peeled and sliced lengthwise

Thin jalapeno chili slices

2 tablespoons chopped unsalted peanuts, toasted

2 lime wedges

Directions:

Heat a pan over medium-high Heat 1 tablespoon of the oil in the pan. Add tempeh and cook until very crisp and browned, takes about 2 minutes per side. Transfer to a plate. Combine the soy sauce, vinegar, salt, 1 tablespoon of the cilantro, and the remaining sesame oil in a bowl. Add the Brussels sprouts, and mix to coat.

Divide between 2 bowls. Sprinkle with jalapeno chili slices and peanuts, and top with the tempeh slices. Pour the remaining dressing, and top with the remaining cilantro. Serve with lime wedges.

Vegetarian Creamy Spaghetti Carbonara

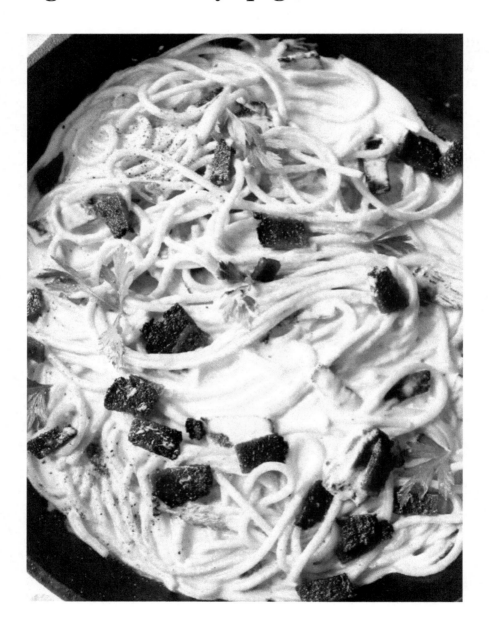

Ingredients

<u>Cashew Sauce:</u>

1 cup of cashews (soaked overnight)

3/4 cup vegetable broth

¼ cup heavy cream

¼ cup shredded mozzarella

4 cloves of garlic minced

1 red onion minced

<u>Sea salt Pepper Carbonara:</u>

250 g whole-wheat spaghetti pasta

300 g white close cup mushrooms (sliced)

1 cup green peas (fresh or frozen)

1 small red onion (minced)

3 clove garlic (minced)

1- 2 tbsp extra-virgin olive oil

fresh parsley

Sea salt Black pepper

Directions:

<u>To Make The Cashew Cheese</u>

Wash the cashews and process in a blender with the rest of ingredients. Blend until you have smooth texture.

To Make The Spaghetti Carbonara

Cook your pasta according to the package instructions. Drizzle with olive oil. Heat olive oil in a pan with medium heat. Add garlic and stir fry for 1 minute. Add onion and mushrooms and stir fry until brown (for about 5 mins.). Add peas and cook further for 3 mins. Stir in ¼ cup of cashew cheese Garnish with fresh parsley.

Quinoa with Pesto Cream

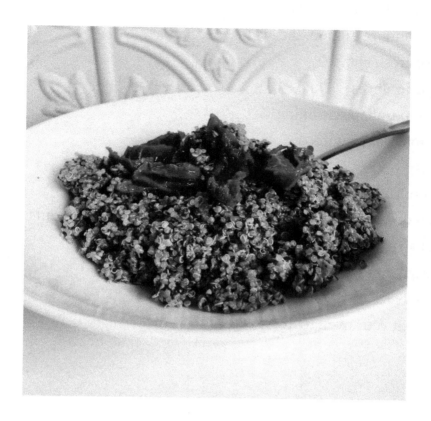

Ingredients

<u>Pesto Cream</u>

2 large bunches basil (about 2 cups lightly packed leaves)

1/4 cup extra virgin olive oil

1/4 cup cream

1 garlic clove 1 tsp pecorino romano cheese

Sea salt and pepper to taste

Quinoa Filling

1 tbsp extra virgin olive oil

1 medium red onion, diced

10 oz fresh spinach

3 garlic cloves

1/2 tsp Italian seasoning

3 cups cooked quinoa

6 tbsp vegan pesto

Sea salt Black pepper to taste

Tomatoes - 6 large tomatoes, (seeds and cores scooped out)

2 Tbsp extra virgin olive oil

Sea salt and pepper to taste

fresh basil

Preheat your oven to 400 degrees F.

Directions:

Combine all of the pesto ingredients in a blender and blend until smooth. In a pan, sauté the onion in olive oil for 7 minutes or until translucent. Add the spinach and garlic cloves and cook for 2 more minutes. Add the cooked quinoa, pesto sauce, Italian seasonings, salt, and pepper. Cut the top of each tomatoes. Scoop out all the seeds. Drizzle olive oil in a baking pan and spread it around.

Place the tomatoes in the baking pan and drizzle with a tbsp of oil over the top of the tomatoes. Season with salt & pepper. Ladle the pesto Quinoa Filling into each of the tomatoes and put the tops back on. Roast for 30 minutes. Garnish with basil.

Southeast Asian Fried Rice

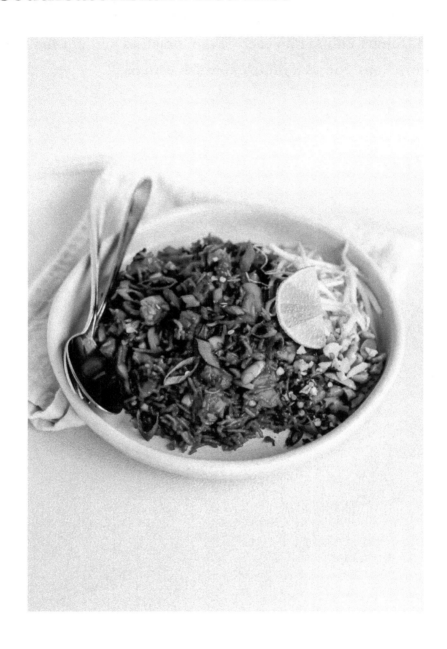

Ingredients

1 cup raw short grain rice

1 red onion, chopped

6 cloves of garlic, chopped

1 tablespoon olive oil

2 carrots, cut into thin sticks

1/2 green bell pepper, cut into thin sticks

1/2 cup frozen peas

1/2 cup cashews

1 tablespoon soy sauce

1 tablespoon red curry powder

1 cup pineapple, cut into small pieces

2 green onions, cut into rings

Sea salt, to taste

black pepper, to taste

red pepper flakes

fresh cilantro (optional)

Cook the rice according to package instructions. Cook the peas for 7 minutes.

Directions:

Heat the oil in a pan and cook the onion for about 3 minutes. Add the garlic, the carrots, and the bell pepper and cook for 3 minutes.

Add the rice and season with curry powder and the soy sauce. Add the pineapple, the peas, the green onion, and cashews. Sprinkle with salt, black pepper, and if using red pepper flakes.

Vegetarian Spaghetti

Ingredients

9 oz spaghetti

1/2 small zucchini, cut into medium-sized pieces

1/2 small eggplant, cut into medium-sized pieces

1 green bell pepper, cut into medium-sized chunks

1 red onion, chopped

3 cloves of garlic, minced

1 cup cherry tomatoes, cut into halves

1/2 cup broccoli, cut into florets

1 handful kale, roughly chopped

3 1/2 cup vegetable stock

1 teaspoon dried Italian herbs (I used thyme, basil, rosemary, and oregano)

salt

black pepper

Directions:

Place all ingredients in a pot except for the kale and the broccoli florets. Pour in the vegetable stock. Season with dried herbs, sea salt, and pepper. Cook for about 13 ½ minutes or until the pasta is al dente (tender but has some firmness to the bite). Add kale and the broccoli 9 minutes after cooking.

Curried Lima Beans

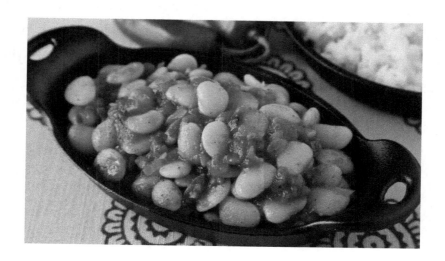

Ingredients

2 Tbsp extra virgin olive oil

1 medium red onion , diced

4 cloves garlic, minced

2 15 oz can lima beans, drained

1 20 oz can tomato sauce

1 cup water

1 Tbsp red curry powder

1/2 bunch fresh cilantro , rinsed and stems removed and coarsely chopped

Stir fry the onion and garlic in a pan with olive oil over medium heat until softened (takes about 4 minutes).

Directions:

Drain the beans and add to the pan. Add the tomato sauce, water and curry powder. Stir everything is well-mixed. Simmer over medium heat. Add cilantro to the pot. Stir and simmer until the sauce has a thick consistency.

Kale and Quorn Pesto Salad

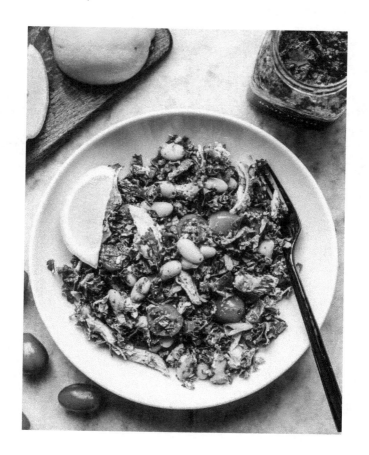

Ingredients

6 cups kale, finely chopped

15 oz. can borlotti beans, rinsed and drained

1 cup cooked quorn*, chopped

1 cup grape tomatoes, sliced in half

1/2 cup pesto

1 large lemon, cut into wedges

Directions:

Combine all of the ingredients in a bowl except for the pesto and lemon Add the pesto and toss until coated.

Vegetarian Tofu Wrap

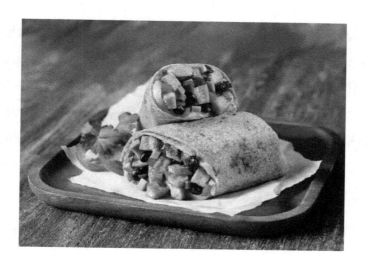

Ingredients

½ red cabbage, shredded

4 heaped tbsp dairy-free yogurt

3 tbsp mint sauce

3 x 7 ounce packs tofu, each cut into 15 cubes

2 Tbsp tandoori curry paste

2 Tbsp extra virgin olive oil

2 red onions, sliced

2 large garlic cloves, sliced

8 chapattis

2 limes, cut into quarters

Directions:

Combine the cabbage, dairy-free yogurt and mint sauce in a bowl. Season with salt and pepper and set aside. Combine the tofu, tandoori paste and 1 Tbsp of the oil. Heat oil on a pan and cook the tofu in batches until golden. Take the tofu off the pan. Add the remaining oil, stir fry the onions and garlic, and cook for 9 mins . Return the tofu to the pan Add more salt. To Assemble Warm the chapattis following package instructions. Top each one with cabbage, tofu and a squeeze of lime juice.

Vegetarian Navy Bean Chili

Ingredients

2 Tbsp extra virgin olive oil 6 garlic cloves, finely chopped

2 large red onions, chopped

3 tbsp sweet pimenton or mild chili powder

3 tbsp ground cumin

Sea salt, to taste

3 tbsp cider vinegar

2 Tbsp honey

2 (14 oz.) cans chopped tomatoes

2 (14 oz.) cans navy beans, rinsed and drained

For garnishing:

crumbled vegan cheese, chopped spring onions, sliced radishes, avocado chunks, soured cream

Directions:

Heat the olive oil and fry the garlic and onions for until softened. Stir in the pimenton and cumin, cook for 3 mins, Add the vinegar, honey, tomatoes and sea salt.

Cook for 10 more mins. Add the beans and cook for another 10 mins. Serve with rice and sprinkle with the garnishing ingredients.

Lima Bean and Pea Salad

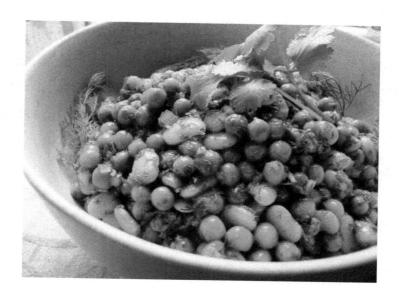

Ingredients

½ cup extra virgin olive oil

1 Tbsp garam masala

2 (14 oz.) cans lima beans, drained and rinsed

½ pound ready-to-eat mixed grain pouch

½ pound frozen peas

2 lemons, zested and juiced

1 large pack parsley, leaves roughly chopped

1 large mint leaves, roughly chopped

Half pound radishes, roughly chopped

1 cucumber, chopped

pomegranate seeds, to serve

Directions:

Preheat your oven to 392 degrees F. Add ¼ cup oil with the garam masala and add some salt. Combine this with the chickpeas in a large roasting pan then cook for 15 mins. or until crisp. Add the mixed grains, peas and lemon zest. Stir and return to the oven for about 10 mins. Toss with the herbs, radishes, cucumber, remaining oil and lemon juice. Season with more salt and garnish with the pomegranate seeds.

Broccoli & Basmati Rice Pilaf

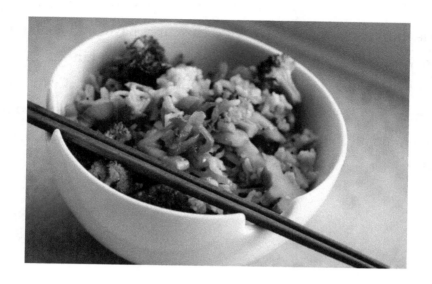

Ingredients

1 tbsp olive oil

2 large red onions, sliced

1 Tbsp curry paste of your choice

½ pound basmati rice

¾ pound broccoli florets

1 pound chickpeas, rinsed and drained

2 cups vegetable stock

1/8 cup toasted flaked almonds

handful chopped coriander

Directions:

Heat the oil in a pan and cook the onions over medium heat for 5 mins until it starts to brown. Add the curry paste and cook for 1 min. Add in the rice, broccoli and chickpeas. Combine all of this to coat. Add in the stock and combine thoroughly. Cover and simmer for 12 ½ mins or until the rice and broccoli become tender and all the liquid has been reduced. Add the almonds and coriander.

Avocado Pasta

Ingredients

2 avocados, pitted and diced

3 cloves garlic, minced

Juice of 1/2 lemon

1/4 cup unsweetened almond milk

1/4 cup water

Sea salt, to taste

Red pepper flakes, to taste

4 halved cherry tomatoes as garnish (optional)

2 cups cooked fettucini

Directions:

Mix the avocados, garlic, and lemon juice in a blender. Slowly add the almond milk and water to the mixture. Add sea salt and red pepper flakes. Toss with your cooked pasta.

Vegetarian Quorn Salad

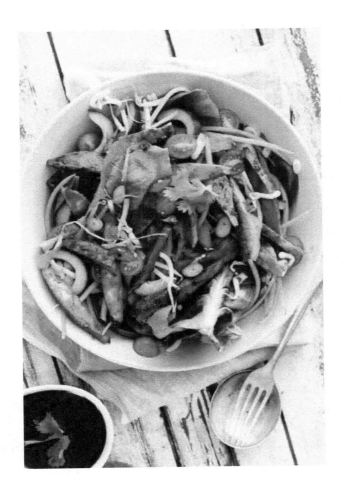

Ingredients

16 oz. quorn, cooked

2 tsp. fresh lemon Juice

1 stalk celery, diced

1/3 cup minced green onions

1 cup mayonnaise

1 tsp. dijon mustard

Sea salt and pepper, to taste

Directions:

Mix the quorn lemon juice, celery, and onions thoroughly. Add the vegan mayonnaise and the mustard to this mixture. Season with sea salt and pepper. Chill and serve.

Mexican Spaghettini Soup

Ingredients

5 large tomatoes, cut into large cubes

1 medium red onion, cut into large cubes

3 cloves garlic

2 Tbsp. olive oil

16 oz. spaghettini, broken into 1-inch pieces

32 oz. vegetable broth

1/2 tsp. Sea salt

1/2 Tbsp. black pepper

2 Tbsp. oregano

2 Tbsp. cumin Chili flakes, chopped

Serrano chilies, or diced jalapeños, to taste (optional)

Directions:

Cilantro, soy sour cream, and sliced avocado, for garnish (optional) Puree the tomatoes, red onions, garlic, and oil. Transfer to a and cook on medium heat. Add in the noodles, broth, salt, pepper, oregano, and cumin. Add the chili flakes, Serrano chilies. Cook for 13 ½ minutes and simmer until the noodles become tender. Garnish with cilantro, soy sour cream or avocado.

Blueberry and Kale Citrus Salad

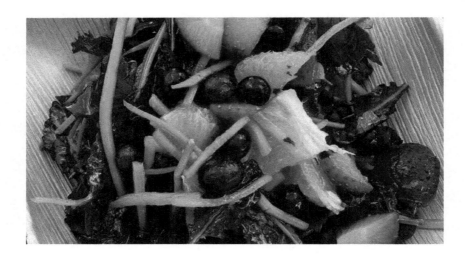

Ingredients

1 bunch kale, stemmed and torn to bite sized pieces 1 lb.
blueberries, sliced

1/4 cup sliced almonds

<u>Dressing Ingredients</u>

Juice of 1 lemon

3 tbsp. extra virgin olive oil

1 Tbsp. honey

1/8 tsp. Sea salt

1/8 tsp. white pepper

3-4 Tbsp. orange juice

In a bowl combine the kale, strawberries and almonds.

Directions:

Combine all of the dressing ingredients and pour over the salad.
Makes 3 to 4 servings

Spinach Stir Fry

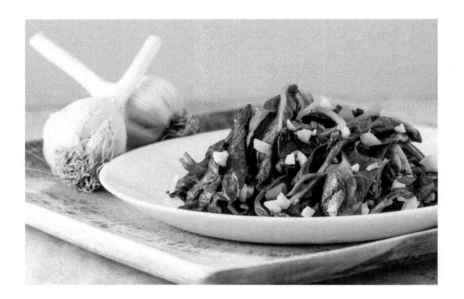

Ingredients

1 package firm spinach, rinsed and drained

Juice of 1/2 lemon

1/2 tsp. salt

1/2 tsp. turmeric

1 Tbsp. olive oil

1/4 cup diced green pepper

1/4 cup diced red onion

3 clove garlic, minced

1 Tbsp. chopped flat-leaf parsley

1 Tbsp. vegan bacon bits (optional)

Pepper, to taste (optional)

Directions:

In a bowl, mix the spinach, lemon juice, salt, and turmeric thoroughly. Heat the oil over medium heat and add the pepper, onion, and garlic. Stir fry for 2 1/2 minutes, or until just softened. Add the tofu mixture and cook for 15 minutes. Garnish with the parsley the soy bacon pieces and pepper.

Easy Kale Stir Fry

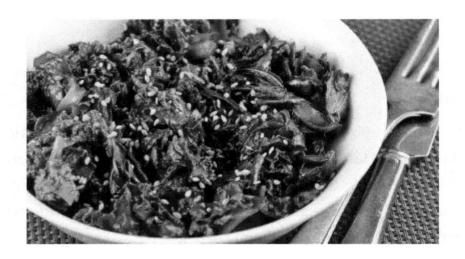

Ingredients

1 package firm kale, rinsed and drained ½ tsp. vinegar

1/2 tsp. salt

1 Tbsp. sesame oil

1/4 cup diced green pepper

1/4 cup diced red onion

3 clove garlic, minced

1 Tbsp. chopped flat-leaf parsley

1 Tbsp. vegan bacon bits (optional)

Pepper, to taste (optional)

In a bowl, mix the kale, vinegar, and salt thoroughly.

Directions:

Heat the oil over medium heat and add the pepper, onion, and garlic. Stir fry for 2 1/2 minutes, or until just softened. Add the tofu mixture and cook for 15 minutes. Garnish with the parsley, the soy bacon pieces and pepper.

Choy Sum Stir Fry

Ingredients

1 bunch choy sum, rinsed and drained

1/2 tsp. Sea salt

1 Tbsp. sesame oil

1/4 cup diced green pepper

1/4 cup diced red onion

3 clove garlic, minced

1 Tbsp. chopped flat-leaf parsley

Pepper, to taste (optional)

In a bowl, mix the choy sum & salt thoroughly.

Directions:

Heat the oil over medium heat and add the pepper, onion, and garlic. Stir fry for 2 1/2 minutes, or until just softened. Add the tofu mixture and cook for 15 minutes. Garnish with the parsley and pepper.

Vegetarian Stuffed Crust Pizza

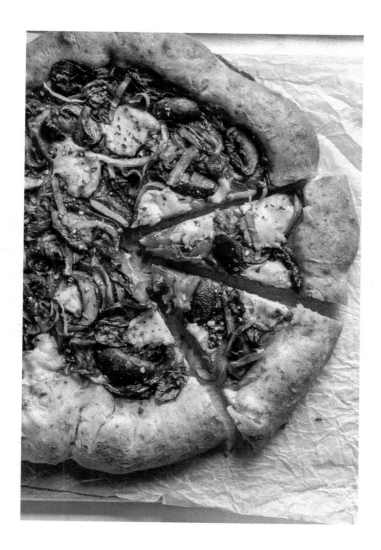

Ingredients

1 box pizza dough (or make your own)

1 block mozzarella, cut into strips

1/3 cup tomato sauce

1 medium tomato, thinly sliced

3 fresh basil leaves, coarsely chopped and dipped in olive oil

1 Tbsp. extra virgin olive oil

Sea salt

Directions:

Preheat your oven to 450°. Stretch out the pizza dough to your desired thickness and place on a lightly oiled and floured baking sheet. Place the vegan mozzarella around the edges of the pizza and roll the edges of the dough up over each strip and press down to make a pocket of cheese. Shred the remaining mozzarella. Spread the pizza sauce over the dough and sprinkle with the shredded vegan cheese. Garnish with the slices of tomato, salt and basil leaves. Bake for 20 minutes, or until the crust is nicely browned.

Avocado and Lima Bean Salad Sandwich

Ingredients

1 15-oz. can lima beans, rinsed, drained, and skinned

1 large, ripe avocado

1/4 cup chopped fresh cilantro

2 Tbsp. chopped green onions

Juice of 1 lime

Sea salt and pepper, to taste

Bread of your choice

Directions:

Lettuce Tomato Mash the lima beans and avocado with a fork. Add cilantro, green onions, and lime juice and stir Season with salt and pepper. Spread on your favorite bread and garnish with lettuce and tomato

Roasted Cauliflower and Garbanzo Beans

Ingredients

cooking spray

1 tablespoon extra virgin olive oil

3 cloves garlic, minced

1/2 teaspoon

Sea salt

1/4 teaspoon ground black pepper

3 1/2 cups sliced cauliflower

2 1/2 cups grape tomatoes

1 (15 ounce) can garbanzo beans, drained

1 lime, cut into wedges

1 tablespoon chopped fresh cilantro

Directions:

Preheat your oven to 450 degrees F. Line a baking sheet with foil and grease with olive oil. Mix the olive oil, garlic, salt, and pepper in a bowl. Add in the cauliflower, tomatoes, and garbanzo beans Combine until well coated. Spread them out in a single layer on the baking sheet. Add the lime wedges. Roast in the oven until vegetables become caramelized, for about 25 minutes. Take out the lime wedges and top with the cilantro.

Roasted Tomato Broccoli and Chickpeas

Ingredients

cooking spray

1 tablespoon extra virgin olive oil

5 cloves garlic, minced

1/2 teaspoon Sea salt

1/4 teaspoon ground black pepper

3 1/2 cups sliced broccoli

2 1/2 cups grape tomatoes

½ tsp. annatto seeds

½ cup green olives

½ cup capers

1 (15 ounce) can chick peas, drained

1 lime, cut into wedges

1 tablespoon chopped fresh cilantro

Directions:

Preheat your oven to 450 degrees F. Line a baking sheet with foil and grease with olive oil. Mix the olive oil, garlic, annatto seeds, salt, and pepper in a bowl. Add in the broccoli, capers, olives, tomatoes, and garbanzo beans Combine until well coated. Spread them out in a single layer on the baking sheet. Add the lime wedges. Roast in the oven until vegetables become caramelized, for about 25 minutes. Take out the lime wedges and top with the cilantro.

Roasted Soybean and Broccoli

Ingredients

cooking spray

1 tablespoon extra virgin olive oil

3 cloves garlic, minced

1/2 teaspoon Sea salt

1/4 teaspoon ground black pepper

3 1/2 cups sliced cauliflower

2 1/2 cups cherry broccoli

1 (15 ounce) can soy beans, drained

1 tsp. cumin

1 tsp. dried annatto seeds

1 tablespoon chopped fresh cilantro

Directions:

Preheat your oven to 450 degrees F. Line a baking sheet with foil and grease with olive oil. Mix the olive oil, garlic, salt, and pepper in a bowl. Add in the cauliflower, broccoli, and soy beans Combine until well coated. Spread them out in a single layer on the baking sheet. Season with cumin. Annatto seeds and more salt if necessary. Roast in the oven until vegetables become caramelized, for about 25 minutes. Take out the lime wedges and top with the cilantro.

Buttery Roasted Tomatoes and Edamame Beans

Ingredients

cooking spray

1 tablespoon melted butter

8 cloves garlic, minced

1/2 teaspoon Sea salt

1/4 teaspoon Italian seasoning

3 1/2 cups sliced cauliflower

2 1/2 cups cherry tomatoes

1 (15 ounce) can edamame beans, drained

1 lime, cut into wedges

¼ cup green olives

Directions:

Preheat your oven to 450 degrees F. Line a baking sheet with foil and grease with olive oil. Mix the olive oil, garlic, salt, and Italian seasoning in a bowl. Add in the cauliflower, green olives, tomatoes, and edamame beans Combine until well coated. Spread them out in a single layer on the baking sheet. Add the lime wedges. Roast in the oven until vegetables become caramelized, for about 25 minutes. Take out the lime wedges and top with the cilantro.

Roasted Choy Sum and Button Mushroom

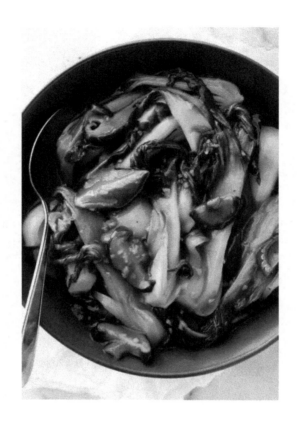

Ingredients

cooking spray

1 tablespoon sesame oil

3 cloves garlic, minced

1/2 teaspoon Sea salt

1/4 teaspoon ground black pepper

3 1/2 cups sliced choy sum

2 1/2 cups sliced button mushrooms

1 tablespoon chopped fresh cilantro

Directions:

Preheat your oven to 450 degrees F. Line a baking sheet with foil and grease with sesame oil. Mix the olive oil, garlic, salt, and pepper in a bowl. Add in the choy sum and button mushrooms Combine until well coated. Spread them out in a single layer on the baking sheet. Add the lime wedges. Roast in the oven until vegetables become caramelized, for about 25 minutes. Top with the cilantro.

Simple Roasted Mustard Greens

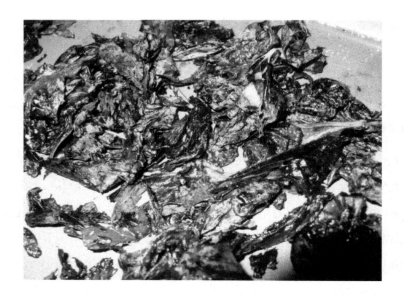

Ingredients

cooking spray

1 tablespoon extra virgin olive oil

3 cloves garlic, minced

1/2 teaspoon Sea salt

1/4 teaspoon ground black pepper

3 1/2 cups sliced mustard greens

2 1/2 cups cherry tomatoes

1 tablespoon chopped fresh thyme

Directions:

Preheat your oven to 450 degrees F. Line a baking sheet with foil and grease with olive oil. Mix the olive oil, garlic, salt, and pepper in a bowl. Add in the mustard greens and tomatoes Combine until well coated. Spread them out in a single layer on the baking sheet. Roast in the oven until vegetables become caramelized, for about 25 minutes. Top with the thyme.

Roasted Mustard Greens and Red Cabbage Extra

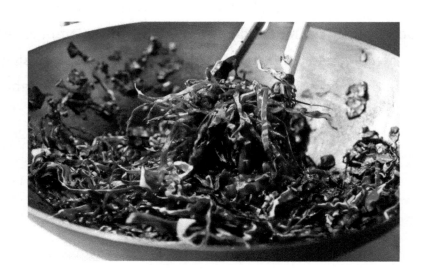

Ingredients

cooking spray

1 tablespoon extra virgin olive oil

1/2 teaspoon Sea salt

1/4 teaspoon ground black pepper

<u>Main Ingredients</u>

1/4 lb. mustard greens

1/2 medium red cabbage, sliced thinly

Directions:

Preheat your oven to 450 degrees F. Line a baking sheet with foil and grease with olive oil. Mix the extra ingredients thoroughly. Add in the main ingredients Combine until well coated. Spread them out in a single layer on the baking sheet. Roast in the oven until vegetables become caramelized, for about 25 minutes.

Roasted Spinach and Artichoke Hearts Extra

Ingredients

cooking spray

1 tablespoon extra virgin olive oil

1/2 teaspoon Sea salt

1/4 teaspoon ground black pepper

Main Ingredients

1 bunch of spinach, rinsed and drained

1 cup canned artichoke hearts

Directions:

Preheat your oven to 450 degrees F. Line a baking sheet with foil and grease with olive oil. Mix the extra ingredients thoroughly. Add in the main ingredients Combine until well coated. Spread them out in a single layer on the baking sheet. Roast in the oven until vegetables become caramelized, for about 25 minutes.

Roasted Parsnips and Watercress Extra

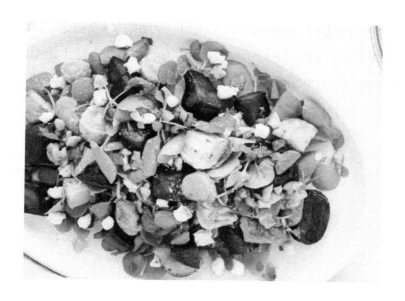

Ingredients

cooking spray

1 tablespoon extra virgin olive oil

1/2 teaspoon Sea salt

1/4 teaspoon ground black pepper

<u>Main Ingredients</u>

1 medium parsnip, sliced thinly

1 bunch of watercress, rinsed and drained

Directions:

Preheat your oven to 450 degrees F. Line a baking sheet with foil and grease with olive oil. Mix the extra ingredients thoroughly. Add in the main ingredients Combine until well coated. Spread them out in a single layer on the baking sheet. Roast in the oven until vegetables become caramelized, for about 25 minutes.

Roasted Napa Cabbage Baby Carrots and Watercress Extra

Ingredients

cooking spray

1 tablespoon extra virgin olive oil

1/2 teaspoon Sea salt

1/4 teaspoon ground black pepper

Main Ingredients

1/2 medium Napa cabbage, sliced thinly

5 baby carrots

1 bunch of watercress, rinsed and drained

Directions:

Preheat your oven to 450 degrees F. Line a baking sheet with foil and grease with olive oil. Mix the extra ingredients thoroughly. Add in the main ingredients Combine until well coated. Spread them out in a single layer on the baking sheet. Roast in the oven until vegetables become caramelized, for about 25 minutes.

Roasted Artichoke Hearts and Napa Cabbage Extra

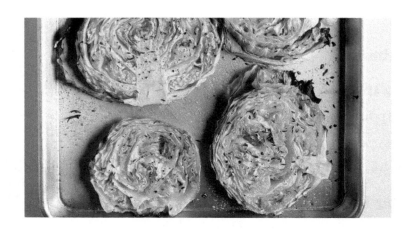

Ingredients

cooking spray

1 tablespoon extra virgin olive oil

1/2 teaspoon Sea salt

1/4 teaspoon ground black pepper

<u>Main Ingredients</u>

1/2 medium napa cabbage, sliced thinly

1 cup canned artichoke hearts

Directions:

Preheat your oven to 450 degrees F. Line a baking sheet with foil and grease with olive oil. Mix the extra ingredients thoroughly. Add in the main ingredients Combine until well coated. Spread them out in a single layer on the baking sheet. Roast in the oven until vegetables become caramelized, for about 25 minutes.

Lightning Source UK Ltd.
Milton Keynes UK
UKHW020702200521
384048UK00001B/33